北京协和医院护理丛书

北京协和医院门诊护理英语

Nursing English in Outpatient Clinics, PUMCH

主编　李　静　吴　宣　宫琦玮

中国协和医科大学出版社
北　京

图书在版编目（CIP）数据

北京协和医院门诊护理英语：汉英对照／李静，吴宣，宫琦玮主编 . — 北京：中国协和医科大学出版社，2020. 12

（北京协和医院护理丛书）

ISBN 978 – 7 – 5679 – 1297 – 7

Ⅰ.①北… Ⅱ.①李… ②吴… ③宫… Ⅲ.①医学 – 英语 Ⅳ.①R

中国版本图书馆 CIP 数据核字（2019）第 102486 号

北京协和医院门诊护理英语
Nursing English in Outpatient Clinic，PUMCH

主　　编：李　静　吴　宣　宫琦玮
责任编辑：王朝霞

出版发行：**中国协和医科大学出版社**
（北京市东城区东单三条9号　邮编100730　电话010 – 65260431）
网　　址：www. pumcp. com
经　　销：新华书店总店北京发行所
印　　刷：北京玺诚印务有限公司

开　　本：787 × 1092　　1/32
印　　张：3. 875
字　　数：22 千字
版　　次：2020 年 12 月第 1 版
印　　次：2020 年 12 月第 1 次印刷
定　　价：42. 00 元

ISBN 978 – 7 – 5679 – 1297 – 7

主　　编　李　静　吴　宣　宫琦玮

副 主 编　丁珊珊　马盼盼　霍静怡

编　　委　（按姓氏笔画为序）

　　　　　马　欣　马睿敏　王　威

　　　　　王　爽　王雪晴　王雅婷

　　　　　王楚涵　甘　泠　卢金鑫

　　　　　刘雨薇　汤有佳　汤　婷

　　　　　李加尧　李秀瑗　何　娜

　　　　　沙京梅　张晓巍　陈　娟

　　　　　罗虹辉　胡盈盈　崔颖颖

　　　　　董　雪　蔡　文

插　　图：于令音　王雨菲

校　　译：陈　茹　王楚涵

前　言

自改革开放以来，随着中国经济的快速发展及国际化进程的不断加快，越来越多的外籍人士选择来华求学或就业。为了充分保障外籍人士的就医，提高医护人员英语水平就显得非常重要。护理人员是医疗服务行业的重要群体，也是患者就诊过程中接触最多的人员。门诊作为患者就医的第一站，该区域里的护理人员英语交流水平直接影响到外籍患者的就医感受。本书以北京协和医院国际医疗部（简称为"协和国际部"）为例，整理、翻译了门诊护士在日常工作中的常用语，以期供其他护理人员参考、借鉴。

本书将门诊护理常用语分为"分诊""治疗""预约""注意事项"四章，每一章又分为若干小结，涵盖了门诊服务的方方面面，如第二章"治疗"中，从抽血、测心电图、测血压到产科、妇科、眼科等专科巡诊，门诊护士常用语都包含其中。本书中文由协和国际部门诊护士们利用工作之余整理汇总，英文译文则由协和国际部英语专业行政人员初译，由经验丰富的高年资护士多次复审、修改，前后耗时近两年，力求内容高品质，同时兼具实用性和准确性。

本书适合在工作中需要跟外籍患者沟通的医护人员借鉴学习，也欢迎其他医疗相关服务行业人员参考。因为能力有限，书中出现缺陷和错误在所难免，欢迎批评指正。

编者

2019 年 9 月

目 录

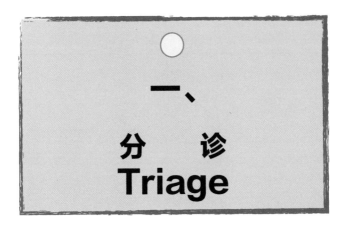

一、

分　　诊
Triage

1. 请问您预约了吗？

   Have you made an appointment?

2. 请问您挂号了吗？

   Have you registered?

3. 请问您交费了吗？

   Have you paid the fee?

4. 请问您有就诊卡吗？

   Do you have a Hospital ID Card/Registration Card?

5. 请您在 5 诊室就诊。

   Please go to Consulting Room 5 and see your doctor there.

6. 5 诊室在左手边第 2 间。

   Consulting Room 5 is the second room on your left hand.

7. 请问您有病历本吗？

   Do you have a Medical Record Booklet?

8. 给您一个病历本。

   Here is a Medical Record Booklet for you.

9. 您是第一次来我们医院就诊吗？

   Is this your first time to see a doctor here?

10. 您需要提前预约。

    You need to make an appointment in advance.

11. 您预约了哪位医生呀？

Which doctor did you make an appointment with?

12. 您约的是几点呀？

What time is your appointment?

13. 您的特约医生是 xx 医生。

You made a specialist appointment with Dr. XX.

14. 我给 xx 医生打电话。

I will call Dr. XX for you.

15. xx 医生在手术，请稍等。

Dr. XX is conducting an operation now, please wait for a while.

16. 稍等，我们给您取病历。

Please wait a second. We will get your medical record booklet here.

17. 请到第二个窗口交费取号。

Please pay the registration fee and get your registration note at the second window.

18. 请到收费窗口挂号。

Please register at the Cashier.

19. 妇产科在一层。

Obstetrics and Gynecology clinic is on the first

floor.

20. 内科在三层就诊。

The Internal Medicine clinic is on the third floor.

21. 右手拐弯坐电梯到一层。

Please turn right and take the elevator to the first floor.

22. X 线室在二层。

X-ray Room is on the second floor.

23. 请用有效证件办理就诊卡。

Please apply for a Hospital ID card with your valid ID.

24. 交费后请到药房取药。

Please pay the fee and then get your medicine at the Pharmacy.

25. 您哪里不舒服？

How do you feel?

What seems to be the problem with you?

What's troubling you?

26. 受伤过久了，需要看骨科。

After having been injured for such a long time, you need to see an orthopedist first.

27. 您发烧吗？

Do you have a fever?

28. 先测量一下您的血压。

I'm going to take your blood pressure first.

29. 我先量一下您的体温。

I'm going to take your temperature first.

30. 我先量一下您的体重。

I'm going to take your weight first.

31. 您需要建个大病历。

You need to apply for a Medical Record.

We are going to set up a medical file for you.

32. 医生开了住院单了吗?

Has your doctor issued a hospitalization admission certificate for you?

33. 我帮您联系一下医生。

I will contact your doctor for you.

34. 您发烧了，需要去发热门诊就诊。

You have got a fever. Please go to the Fever Clinic to see a doctor.

35. 您先到取血室抽血。

Please take a blood test in the Blood Drawing Room.

Please go to the Blood Drawing Room and we are going to take some blood samples for you.

36. 让我看看您都有哪些检查。

    Please let me see what blood tests need to be performed.

37. 您需要抽血。

    You need to take a blood test.

38. 抽血室在二层大门口旁，右手第一间。

    Blood Drawing Room is on the second floor, next to the main entrance, on your right hand.

39. 您需要做心电图。

    You need to take an ECG/EKG.

40. 心电图在二层治疗室做。

    ECG room is on the second floor.

41. 您需要做 B 超检查。

    You need to take an ultrasound examination.

42. 我先给您排个序号。

    Let me help you to get a sequence number.

43. 超声诊断室在您身后。

    Ultrasound Room is behind you.

44. 您需要照个胸片，X 线室在二层西侧。

    You need to take an X-ray upon your chest. X-ray Room is in the west side of the second floor.

45. 医生预约您下一次复诊了吗?

Has your doctor made an appointment for your return visit?

46. 您需要定期来检查。

You need to take a regular visit.

47. 如果您觉得更严重了，马上过来医院就诊。

If your symptom gets worse, please come to the hospital immediately.

48. 如果您觉得不舒服，请马上来医院。

If you feel sick, please come to the hospital right away.

49. 医生给您开了一个疗程的药。

The doctor prescribed a course of medicine for you.

50. 明天早上空腹来抽血。

Please come to take a fasting blood test tomorrow morning.

51. xx 会在诊断证明书上给您盖章。

XX will stamp your diagnosis certificate.

52. 医生让您做一个全血检查。

The doctor asked you to take a full blood count test.

53. 需要我再解释一下吗？

Do you need me to explain it again for you?

54. 医生让您休息几天。

The doctor asked you to take a rest for several days.

55. 医生让您拍张 X 线片确认一下。

The doctor asked you to take an X-ray for confirmation.

56. 医生让您住院观察。

The doctor asked you to be hospitalized for observation.

57. 我来帮您办理住院手续。

Let me help you to get the hospitalization procedures done.

58. 医生说不严重。

The doctor said it's not severe.

59. 您以前来过这里看病吗?

Have you seen a doctor here before?

60. 您带就诊卡了吗?

Do you bring your Hospital ID Card?

61. 您应该先看皮科,需要的话再看变态反应科。

Firstly, you should see a dermatologist, then you can see an allergist if needed.

62. 每次来看病,记得带就诊卡。

Every time you come to see a doctor here,

please bring your Hospital ID Card.

63. 沿这条路走到药房再向左拐就能看到厕所了。

Go ahead and turn left at the Pharmacy, and then you will see the restroom.

64. 您测量体温了吗？是多少？

Have you taken your temperature? What is it?

65. 我帮您联系口腔科医生。

I will help you contact a dentist.

66. 您的牙什么时候肿的？

When did your tooth become swollen up like this?

67. 您最近的一次牙齿检查是什么时候？

When was your last dental check-up?

68. 您最近的一次看牙是什么时候？

When was the last time you saw the dentist?

69. 您最近的一次口腔洁治在什么时候？

When was the last time of your scaling?

70. 您刷牙时牙龈出血吗？

Do your gums bleed when you brush your teeth?

71. 能描述一下您的疼痛感觉吗？

Could you describe what your pain feels like?

72. 疼痛有放射吗？

Does the pain radiate?

73. 您感觉它是钝痛吗？

   Does it feel like a dull pain?

74. 它是锐痛吗？

   Is it a sharp pain?

75. 牙痛是间断地痛吗？

   Does the pain come and go?

76. 您（这颗牙）以前痛过吗？

   Have you ever had a toothache before?

77. 喝冷水时痛吗？

   Do you feel painful when drinking cold water?

78. 喝热水时痛吗？

   Do you feel painful when drinking hot water?

79. 吃甜食时痛吗？

   Do you feel painful when eating sweets?

80. 咬硬物时痛吗？

   Do you feel painful when biting hard things?

81. 夜间疼痛会加重吗？

   Did it hurt more at night?

82. 疼痛有缓解吗？

   Has the toothache been alleviated?

83. 您吃过止痛（镇痛）片吗？

   Have you ever had any painkillers?

84. 这个是心内科专家。

He/She is a cardiologist.

85. 这是医生开的止痛药，建议您现在服用。

This is the pain killer that your doctor prescribed. It is suggested to take it right now.

86. 您能走路吗?

Can you walk?

87. 我们的导医会带您去做检查。

Our hospital guide will lead you to take examinations.

88. 我用轮椅推您走吧。

I will push you with a wheelchair.

89. 国际部就诊医保不报销，但是商业保险可以报销。

You need to pay the full bills at the International Medical Department. But if you have commercial health insurance, you can get reimbursed by your insurance company.

90. 国际部费用只有药费和普通门诊一样，其他费用都高。

The costs in the International Medical Department are higher than General Outpatient Clinic except for the medicine.

91. 商业保险患者在二层商业保险接待处办理相关

手续。

Patients with commercial health insurance please go to Commercial Insurance Reception which is located on the second floor.

92. 病案室在一层东侧。

Medical Records Office is located in the east of the first floor.

93. 洗手间每个楼层都有。

There are restrooms on every floor.

94. 预防接种在一层。

Vaccination room is on the first floor.

95. 预防接种只接收在协和国际部出生和外籍的宝宝接种疫苗。

Vaccination service is only available for the babies born at the International Medical Department or foreign babies.

96. 您有什么全身性疾病吗?

Do you have any systemic diseases?

97. 您有什么慢性病吗?

Do you have any chronic diseases?

98. 您既往有什么病吗?

Could you tell me your past medical history?

二、

治　疗
Treatment

抽血
Blood Drawing

1. 请给我您的就诊卡。

   Please show me your Hospital ID Card.

2. 请卷起袖子，露出胳膊肘正中血管部分。

   Please roll up your sleeve and show the vascular part of your elbow.

3. 您的血液检查需要空腹，请问您是否吃早饭了？

   You need to take a fasting blood test. Did you have breakfast this morning?

4. 给您系好止血带。

   I have tied a tourniquet for you.

   请您握拳。

   Please make a fist.

   抽好血了。

   Blood drawing is done.

   请您松拳，按压穿刺部位 5 分钟。

   Please loosen your fist and press the puncture point for 5 minutes.

5. 请您把衣服穿好。

Please put on your clothes.

6. 请您根据条码上提示的出结果时间，在自助机打印化验单。

You can use the self-service machine to print your blood test results according to the time on your barcode note.

也可以上医院 APP 查询化验结果。

You can also use our official APP to check your test results.

并再次电话预约医生就诊。

Please make another appointment with your doctor by calling us after you get the results.

7. 小宝宝抽血常规和大人有区别。

It's different to draw blood for babies.

小宝宝是需要取指血。

We need to pinch the baby's finger with a needle and then get blood by squeezing the finger.

8. 抱歉，该项血液检查操作不能有家属陪同。

Sorry, family members are not allowed to accompany during this blood test.

请您配合，谢谢。

Thank you for your cooperation.

心电图
Electrocardiography (ECG)

1. 请解开衣服。露出胸前区。

    Please unbutton your clothes and show your chest.

2. 请解开胸罩。

    Please untie your bra.

3. 请平躺在检查床上。

    Please lie flat on your back.

4. 露出双手腕及双脚踝。

    Show your wrists and ankles.

5. 做检查时请保持安静。

    Please keep quiet when taking the examination.

6. 做检查前请先安静休息 10 分钟。

    Please stay quiet and rest for 10 minutes before the examination.

7. 双手自然放在身体两侧。

    Put your hands naturally at both sides of your body.

8. 取结果请咨询护士。

    Please consult our nurses if you want to get your results.

测量血压
Taking Blood Pressure

1. 请休息 10 分钟。

   Please take a rest for 10 minutes.

2. 请伸出左胳膊（或右胳膊）。

   Please stick out your left(right) arm.

3. 请将外衣脱掉。

   Please take off your coat.

4. 衣服袖口不要太紧。

   Please loosen your cuff.

5. 我给您量一下血压。

   I will take your blood pressure.

6. 请正常呼吸。

   Please breathe normally.

7. 请放松，不要紧张。

   Please relax. Don't be nervous.

8. 袖带有点紧。

   The blood pressure cuff is a little tight.

9. 您的血压正常。

   Your blood pressure is normal.

10. 您的血压有点高（或低）。

    Your blood pressure is a little higher (lower).

24 小时动态血压监测
24-hour Dynamic Blood Pressure Monitoring

1. 请问您的出生日期是什么时候？

   Could you tell me your birth date?

2. 我先准备用物。

   I am preparing some articles for the test.

   请您稍等。

   Please wait for a minute.

3. 请和我来，将外衣脱掉，露出胳膊（左右均可）。

   Please come with me, take off your coat and show me your arm (either left or right is OK).

4. 请放松，不要紧张。

   Please relax and don't be nervous.

   我先给您测一次血压。

   I will take your blood pressure first.

   您感受一下袖带是否过紧。

   You can feel whether the blood pressure cuff is too tight.

5. 本次测量血压正常。

   Your blood pressure is normal this time.

6. 那我再帮您调整一下。

Let me help you adjust that a little bit.

7. 今晚不能洗澡。

You can't take a shower or bath this evening.

这个小盒子要一直带着，明天这个时间来摘。

Please carry this small box with you all the time and come to take it off at this time tomorrow.

8. 白天每半小时自动测量一次，夜间每一小时测量一次。

The device will take your blood pressure every half hour during daytime and every hour at night.

测量过程中最好静止放松，夜间避免挤压到检查肢体。

Please stay relaxed when your blood pressure is taken and avoid pressing the monitored arm.

9. 请您稍等，大概 15 分钟后报告会送到您手中。

Please wait. The report will be delivered to you in 15 minutes.

24 小时动态心电图
24-hour Holter Monitoring

1. 您好，请您到治疗室稍等。

Hello, please wait for me in the Treatment Room.

我准备用物，稍后过去为您操作。

I will get prepared and install it for you later.

2. 您好，此项检查和心电图一样要在您胸部粘贴电极片。

Hello. This test is the same as ECG. I need to stick several electrodes on your chest.

请您露出胸部。

Please show me your chest.

3. 已经连接好设备，请您放心。

OK, the device has been connected well.

4. 取下设备前不可洗澡。

Please don't take a shower or bath before this device is taken off.

这个小盒子要挂在您身上。

This small box will be on you all along.

同时避免电极纽扣脱落。

Please avoid dropping any electrode.

若有脱落及时与我们联系。

If any electrode falls off, please contact us immediately.

5. 明日同一时间再来取下这个装置。

Come back at the same time tomorrow to have this device removed.

报告需 3 个工作日后到护士站取。

Please come to take your report at the Nurse Station in three workdays.

取报告时需携带患者本人就诊卡。

When you come to get your report, please bring your Hospital ID Card.

尿标本采集
Urine Specimen Collection

1. 您最好留取清晨第一次尿做检查。

   You'd better collect your early morning urine for examination.

2. 给您尿管及收集器。

   Here is the urine sample tube and container.

   将尿液尿在收集器里，最好是中段尿，再倒入尿管里，大约 8 ~ 10ml。

   Get your midstream urine sample to this container, around 8 ~ 10ml.

3. 这是防腐剂。

   This is the preservative.

4. 请准备一个尿桶。将 24 小时内尿全部尿在这个尿桶里。

Please get a container to collect your urine for the next 24 hours.

5．尿第一次尿后，请将防腐剂倒入尿桶。

After urinating into the container for the first time, pour the preservative inside.

6．请测量整个 24 小时所有尿，记录总量。

Please measure and record the volume of your 24-hour urine.

7．取其中 10ml 留在尿标本瓶内。

Take 10ml from the container and put it into a urine specimen bottle.

8．留 24 小时尿。从清晨第一次尿排掉开始计时，至次日同一个时间。

When taking 24-hour urine test, you should start from urinating for the first time in the morning to the same time of the next day.

9．请把留好的尿交到实验室。

Please bring your urine specimen to the Laboratory.

10．请将尿瓶盖拧紧，以免遗洒。

Please screw the lid to prevent it from spilling.

11．24 小时尿检时，请避开经期。

Please avoid your period when taking the 24-hour urine test.

12. 女病人留尿前，清洁外阴，避免阴道分泌物或白带影响结果。

A female patient should clean her private parts first; otherwise vaginal fluid and leucorrhea will affect the test results.

13. 留清洁中段尿前，需将外阴清洁消毒。

Please clean your private part before taking your midstream urine specimen.

14. 留尿后立即送检。

Please send the urine for test immediately after finishing the collection.

牙科治疗
Dental Treatment

1. 今天医生要给您做补牙治疗。

The doctor will fill your decayed teeth today.

2. 您有 N 个楔状缺损需要填充。

You have N teeth with wedge-shaped defects that need to be filled.

3. 如果您感到疼痛，请举左手。

If you feel pain, please raise your left hand.

4. 橡皮障是为了防止唾液影响治疗。

The rubber dam is designed to prevent saliva from affecting the treatment.

5. 今天要进行根管治疗。

The root canal treatment will be done today.

6. 您的牙髓发炎了。

Your pulp is inflamed.

7. 医生在做根管荡洗。

The dentist is doing the root canal irrigation.

8. 医生用临时材料做了暂时封闭。

The dentist will fill the cavity with some temporary sealing materials.

9. N 周后需要复诊。

You should come back in N weeks.

10. 治疗期间牙齿可能会有异样感。

You may have a strange feeling from your teeth during the treatment.

11. 一周之内您可能会感觉有点痛。

You may feel a little pain this week.

12. 如有必要，医生会给您打麻药。

The dentist will give you an anesthetic injection as needed.

13. 死髓牙的颜色会随时间的推移而改变。

The color of non-vital tooth will change as time

goes on.

14. 这颗牙龋坏很严重。

This tooth is decayed seriously.

15. 医生准备给龋坏的牙做树脂填充。

The dentist is going to fill the cavity with the resin.

16. 吸唾管会吸掉您嘴里多余的水。

The saliva suction tube will suck the excess water from your mouth.

17. 请起身漱口。

Please get up and rinse your mouth.

18. 去腐过程牙齿可能敏感。

The teeth may be sensitive when cleaning the decay.

19. 钻牙的时候您可能感觉有点痛。

You may feel a little pain when the teeth are being drilled.

20. 我给您的嘴角涂些凡士林。

I'll apply some Vaseline to the corner of your mouth to lubricate your lips.

21. 您需要照牙片 / 曲断 /CBCT。

You need to take a dental X-ray/panoramic radiography/CBCT .

22. 您照完牙片后请回到诊室等候。

Please go back to the consulting room after the dental X-ray film is taken.

23. 这是抛光膏的味道。

The taste is from the polishing paste.

24. 这颗牙已经松动了，我们要拔了它。

The tooth is loose and need to be extracted.

25. 这颗智齿位置不正，需要拔除。

The position of this wisdom tooth is abnormal and it needs an extraction.

26. 在急性炎症期的牙齿，我们不能拔除。

The teeth which are in acute inflammatory period can not be extracted.

27. 待症状消失后，我们再拔牙。

We will make a tooth extraction after the symptoms disappear.

28. 医生要给您打麻药了。

The dentist will give you a local anesthetic injection.

29. 医生用激光切开舌系带。

The dentist is using the laser to cut the tongue tie.

30. 为了伤口更好的愈合，要在拔牙窝处缝合一针。

For better wound healing, a suture was done in

the extraction socket.

31. 请咬紧纱球 30 分钟。

Please bite the yarn ball for 30 minutes.

32. 医生把这个脓肿切开了。

The dentist has done an incision of the abscess.

33. 我们在切口里放了引流条。

We have put a drainage strip in the incision.

34. 这块切下来的组织要送病理。

This tissue needs to be sent to Pathology.

35. 拔牙前请不要空腹。

Do not come with an empty stomach before the tooth extraction.

36. 拔牙后 3 个月可进行修复治疗。

The prosthodontic treatment can be done three mouths after tooth extraction.

37. 医生在取模型之前，先给您试试托盘。

The dentist will let you try the tray first before taking your model.

38. 如果感觉义齿有压着牙龈的情况，请复诊，医生会为您调整。

If there is pressure on gums, please come back and the dentist will adjust it for you.

39. 桩核起到支持牙齿的作用。

The core and post play a role in supporting the tooth.

40. 由于患牙非常薄弱，需要放置桩核。

It is necessary to place a core, as the tooth is very weak.

41. 每天晚上将义齿摘下，泡入冷水中。

Take off the denture every evening and soak it in cold water.

42. 义齿不可用酒精或其他药品浸泡。

The denture can not be soaked in alcohol or other drugs.

43. 义齿不可蒸煮消毒。

The denture can not be boiled for disinfection.

44. 正畸治疗可以改善容貌。

The orthodontic treatment can improve one's looks.

45. 正畸治疗可以改善牙齿的功能。

The orthodontic treatment can improve the function of your teeth.

46. 正畸治疗有固定矫治器和活动矫治器矫正牙齿。

There are fixed and removable appliances for the orthodontic treatment.

47. 正畸治疗期间保持牙齿清洁很重要。

It is important to keep your teeth clean during the orthodontic treatment.

48. 请坚持用牙缝刷清洁牙间隙。

Please keep using an interdental brush to clean the intervals of teeth.

49. 最好不要啃硬食物。

It's better not to eat hard food.

50. 最好不要吃黏性大的食物，如年糕。

You'd better not eat very sticky food, such as rice cakes.

儿童牙科治疗
Pedodontics Treatment

1. 孩子要定期进行口腔检查。

A routine oral examination is necessary for children.

2. 口腔里的细菌会吃掉你的牙齿。

The bacteria in the mouth will eat your teeth.

3. 牙洞变大了就感觉痛了。

If the tooth cavity becomes big, you'll feel pain.

4. 医生会很小心地挖掉这些细菌。

The dentist will excavate these bacteria carefully.

5. 今天医生会给你做窝沟封闭。

The dentist will apply a pit and fissure sealant for you today.

6. 今天医生会补上牙齿上的小洞洞。

The dentist will fill up the small holes on the decayed tooth.

7. 我们需把这颗被虫子吃掉的牙齿拔掉。

We need to pull out the tooth eaten by worms (bacteria).

8. 这是吸唾管，吸掉嘴里的水。

This is a suction pipe, which can drain the water out of your mouth.

9. 这是喷水枪，给牙齿洗澡用的。

This is a water spray used to clean your teeth.

10. 今天的治疗一点也不痛。

Today's treatment will not be painful at all.

11. 让我们一起来给牙齿涂上氟保护剂。

Let's paint the teeth with fluoride varnish together.

12. 涂了氟保护剂的牙齿不易生病了。

The teeth coated with a fluoride varnish are not susceptible to illness.

13. 拔掉这颗牙后需要做个间隙保护器。

A space maintainer is required after the tooth is

pulled out.

14. 最好把这颗乳牙保护到替换期。

It's better to protect the baby tooth till the new tooth erupt.

15. 治疗很快要结束了。

The treatment will be over soon. / Almost done.

16. 我们约好一周后再见，好吗？

Let's meet again a week later, OK?

17. 你今天表现非常棒。

You did a great job today.

18. 现在我们一起刷牙好吗？

Now can we brush the teeth together?

19. 医生钻牙的时候，舌头不要动。

Please don't move your tongue when the dentist is drilling on your teeth.

20. 喝完牛奶后记得要漱口。

Remember to rinse your mouth after drinking milk.

21. 医生要给这颗乳牙做个牙冠。

The dentist will make a crown for the baby tooth.

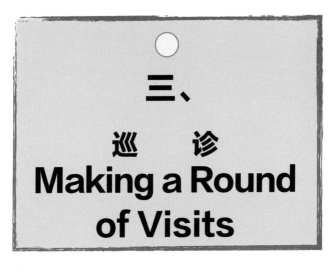

三、

巡　诊
Making a Round
of Visits

1. 请到二楼交费，取药。

   Please go to the second floor to pay the bills and get your medicine.

2. 超声检查请在二层交费后，在护士站排队。

   Please pay the ultrasound test fee on the second floor and take a queue number at the Nurse Station.

3. 请到 N 诊室门口候诊。

   Please wait outside of Consulting Room N.

4. 您已经过号，请在诊室外候诊。

   You missed your turn, please wait outside the Consulting Room.

5. 对不起！您迟到了，医生已经离开了。

   Sorry! You are late and the doctor has left.

6. 您好！有病历本吗?

   Hello! Do you have a Medical Record Booklet?

7. 病历本是免费的。

   This Medical Record Booklet is free.

8. 出口在这边，左手楼梯，右手电梯。

   Exit is over there. The stairs are on your left hand and the elevators on your right hand.

9. 医生已经给您开好住院证，医院会有人与您联系。

   When the doctor issues a hospitalization certificate for you, we will contact you.

10. 您的病历因为很久没有使用，需要大概 1 小时左右才能送来。

   You haven't used your Medical Record for a long time, so it will take around 1 hour to get it to be delivered here.

11. 您想就诊的医生，不在这里出诊，请拨打 xxxxx 特约。

   The doctor you want to consult has no regular outpatient service in our department, but you can call XXXXX for a specialist consulting appointment.

12. 麻醉科医生不需要预约，周一至周五上午 10 点到护士站加号。

   You don't need to make an appointment with an anesthetist. Please go to the Nurse Station at 10:00am from Monday to Friday and ask the nurse to register for you.

13. 请在检查前一周到门诊就诊麻醉科。

   Please consult an anesthetist in our outpatient clinic one week before your examination.

14. 检查结果取出后，请重新预约医生就诊。

   After getting your examination results, please make another appointment with your doctor.

15. 您的检查我们会有专人引领您前往。

We will arrange someone to guide you for your examination.

16. 请到二层交费，然后取血。

Please go to the second floor, pay the fee and have your blood drawn.

17. 退号请到护士站盖章。

If you want to cancel your registration, please go to the Nurse Station and have your registration note stamped.

18. 退费需要您带好交费收据到护士站办理。

If you want to get your fee back, please bring your receipt to the Nurse Station.

19. 心电图检查室在二层。

ECG Room is on the second floor.

20. 请到一层测量体重。

Please go to the first floor to take your weight.

骨科巡诊
Making a Round of Visits in Orthopedics Department

1. 您的腿痛了多久了？

How long has your leg been in pain?

2. 您的腿有外伤吗？

Does your leg have trauma?

3. 您的腰扭了是吗？

Did you hurt your low back ?

4. 您的脚崴了吗？

Did you sprain your ankle?

5. 医生让您先拍 X 线片。

The doctor asked you to take an X-ray first.

6. 医生需要看看您的 X 线片结果。

The doctor needs to have a look at your X-ray result.

7. 您试着走走可以吗？

Can you try to walk?

8. 您需要先请医生帮你正骨。

You need to ask your doctor to manipulate your bones first.

9. 医生先给您包扎一下。

The doctor will bind up your wound first.

10. 您拄着拐杖试着走一下儿。

Please try to walk with this walking stick.

11. 您的手是戳到地上了吗？

Has your hand been stuck to the ground?

12. 医生说您是软组织损伤。

The doctor said that you have soft tissue injury.

13. 把这个药膏抹在伤口上。

Apply this ointment on the wound.

14. 这是止痛药，疼的时候可以吃一片。

These are pain killers. You may take one tablet when you feel painful.

15. 您的伤口很深，医生需要给你缝合。

Your wound is very deep, and the doctor needs to sew up the wound for you.

16. 您会使用三角巾吗？

Can you use a triangle bandage?

17. 您的脚需要制动，不要走路。

Your feet need to rest. Please don't walk.

18. X 线片显示你没有骨折。

X-ray shows that you don't have a fracture.

19. 医生需要您一个星期以后复查。

The doctor asked you to have a re-examination in one week.

20. 您需要去二层打石膏。

You need go to the second floor to wear a cast.

21. 您需要下周来拆线。

You need to come back next week to take out sutures.

22. 您的腿骨折了。

Your leg is broken.

23. 医生让您休息两周。

The doctor asked you to rest for two weeks.

24. 您的脚指头可以动一动吗?

Can you move your toes?

儿科巡诊
Making a Round of Visits in Pediatric Department

1. 宝宝多大了?

How old is your baby?

2. 宝宝发烧吗?

Does your baby/he/she have a fever?

3. 先给宝宝量下体温。

Please take the temperature of your baby.

4. 体温表放在腋下，5分钟后取出。

Put the thermometer under your baby's arm and take it out after 5 minutes.

5. 摸摸额头热吗?

Is his forehead hot?

6. 先给宝宝喝点水吧。

Please feed your baby some water.

7. 宝宝是不是饿了（渴了）？

Is your baby hungry/thirsty?

8. 给宝宝换换尿布。

Please change a diaper for your baby.

9. 隔壁有母乳喂养室。

Breast Feeding Room is next door.

10. 宝宝脚有点凉。

Your baby's feet are a little cold.

11. 宝宝睡着了，请给他／她盖点东西。

Your baby has fallen asleep. Please cover something for him/her.

12. 给宝宝测量体重和身高。

Please take your baby's weight and height.

13. 可以抱着宝宝。

Please hold your baby.

14. 宝宝怎么一直在哭？

Why is your baby crying all the time?

15. 等会儿，医生马上到。

Please wait for a second. The doctor is coming.

16. 宝宝出汗了。

Your baby is sweating.

17. 帮您给宝宝沏点奶吧。

Let me help you make some formula milk for your baby.

18. 宝宝鞋掉了。

The baby's shoe/shoes fell off.

19. 宝宝喝完奶后，请轻拍宝宝的背，以免打嗝。

Please pat the back of your baby to prevent belch when he/she finishes drinking milk.

20. 别着急，下一个就到您就诊了。

Take it easy. You will be next.

21. 这里人多，请照顾好你的孩子，不要让他 / 她到处乱跑。

There are too many people here. Please take care of your kid and don't let him/her run around.

22. 先给宝宝吃退烧药吧。

Please give your baby a fever reducer and it will help him/her to lower the temperature.

23. 宝宝吐奶了，快把他 / 她立起来，拍拍。

The baby spit up milk. You can stand him/her up and pat his/her back.

24. 给宝宝擦擦吧。

Please wipe it for the baby.

25. 宝宝出汗了。

The baby sweats.

26. 宝宝退烧了。

The baby's fever is gone.

27. 宝宝拉稀了。

The baby has a diarrhea.

The baby has loose bowels.

28. 给宝宝化验个大便常规。

We will take a stool routine test for your baby.

29. 医生给您的宝宝开了药。

The doctor prescribed some medicine for your baby.

30. 到前面收费窗口先交费。

Please go to the Cashier over there and pay the bills first.

31. 交费后在旁边的药房取药。

After paying the bills, get the medicine at the Pharmacy nearby.

32. 您取药后我教您如何服用。

After you get the medicine, I will tell you how to take it.

33. 照顾好宝宝。

Take good care of your baby.

34. 宝宝又吐了。

The baby vomited again.

35. 请抱着宝宝在门口坐一会儿。

Please hold your baby and wait outside for a short while.

36. 医生叫您的宝宝就诊。

It's your baby's turn to see the doctor.

37. 您的宝宝需要看皮肤科。

Your baby needs to consult Dermatology.

38. 请带您的孩子去做血常规检查。

Please take your baby for a blood routine test.

39. 宝宝的化验结果出来了。

The test results of your baby have come out.

40. 让医生看看是否正常。

You can ask the doctor to have a look at the results.

41. 宝宝的弟弟也发烧了吗?

Does the baby's litter brother have a fever, too?

42. 如果结果正常，就不用吃药了。

If all the results turn out to be normal, the baby doesn't need to take any medicine.

43. 宝宝知道哪里疼吗?

Does the baby know which part hurts?

44. 这是医生给开的药。

This is the medicine prescribed by the doctor.

45. 一定按时服药。

Please take the medicine on time.

46. 宝宝不能保持太长时间不动，所以我们在拍 X 光片时得抓紧时间。

The baby can't keep still for too long, so we have to hurry when taking an X-ray.

47. 明天早上带宝宝来抽血。

Please take your baby for blood drawing tomorrow morning.

48. 抽血前不要给宝宝吃东西。

Don't feed your baby anything before blood drawing.

49. 不要在宝宝哭闹时试表。

Don't take your baby's temperature when he/ she is crying.

产科巡诊
Making a Round of Visits in Obstetrics Department

1. 您现在怀孕多少周了？

How many weeks have you been pregnant?

2．您怀孕了吗?

Are you pregnant?

3．是用试纸测出怀孕吗?

Did you use test paper to know your pregnancy?

4．您抽过血做化验了吗?

Have you taken blood test?

5．先给您测量血压和体重吧。

Let's take your blood pressure and weight first.

6．每次就诊前都需要测量血压和体重。

We will take your blood pressure and weight every time before you see your doctor.

7．您的血压有点高。

Your blood pressure is a little high.

8．平时血压高吗?

Did you have hypertension before?

9．您休息一会儿再重新测量一次血压。

Please rest for a while and take your blood pressure again later.

10．您现在感觉怎样了?

How do you feel now?

11．您现在感觉好点儿了吗?

Do you feel better now?

12．可以再测量一次血压吗?

Could I take your blood pressure again?

13. 请您脱掉鞋再测体重。

Please take off your shoes before taking your weight.

14. 请站稳不动。

Please stand still.

15. 您的血压是 120/70mmHg。

Your blood pressure is 120/70mmHg.

16. 您的体重是 50kg。

Your weight is 50kg.

17. 下一位就到您了。

You will be the next one.

18. 您办理母子健康手册了吗?

Have you applied for a Mother and Child Health Brochure?

19. 医生会在看诊期间计算您的预产期。

Your doctor will calculate your expected date of childbirth during the consulting.

之后，请到护士站登记床位。

After that please come to the Nurse Station and register for a bed.

20. 您能告诉我您末次月经第一天的日期吗?

Could you please tell me the first day of your

last period?

21. 您能告诉我您的电话吗？

Could you please tell me your phone number?

22. 您能告诉我您的年龄吗？

Could you tell me your age please?

23. 您能告诉我您的国籍吗？

Could you tell me your nationality?

24. 已为您登记好床位。

We have registered a bed for you. / We have made a bed-registration for you.

25. 您今天要做胎心监护吗？

Do you need to take a fetal heart rate monitoring today?

26. 请把您的胎心监护条码给我。

Please give me your barcode of fetal heart rate monitoring.

27. 一会儿有医生为您做监护。

The doctor will come to do the monitoring for you soon.

28. 这是胎心监护结果。

This is the result of your fetal heart rate monitoring.

29. 请交给您的主管医生。

Please give the result to your doctor-in-charge.

30. 医生为什么让您做这个检查呢?

Why did your doctor want you to take this examination?

31. 交费后先抽血。

Please pay the fee first and then take a blood test.

32. B 超是今天做吗?

Have you taken an ultrasound test today?

33. 这个 B 超医生让您过 4 周再做。

Your ultrasound doctor asked you to take this test in four weeks.

34. 先预约好做 B 超的日期。

Please make an appointment for your ultrasound test.

35. 当天持预约条来做 B 超。

Please bring your appointment bar/slip that day to take an ultrasound test.

36. 医生要做检查。

The doctor needs to do the check-up.

37. 这项检查是为了筛查妊娠期糖尿病的。

This exam is to screen gestational diabetes.

38. 检查当日把糖粉交给取血室护士。

On your examination day, please give your sugar powder to the nurse in the Blood Drawing Room.

39. 医生会帮您沏好糖水。

The doctor will make sugar water for you.

40. 抽血前一日晚上 12 点后请不要吃喝任何东西。

Please don't eat or drink anything after 12:00pm the day before your blood drawing day.

41. 抽血当天空腹来。

Please keep fasting on your examination day.

42. 在药房把糖粉取回来。

Please go to the Pharmacy to get your sugar powder.

43. 您可以参加一下我们的准妈妈课堂。

You could attend our classes for expectant mothers.

44. 需要我帮您报名准妈妈课堂吗?

Do you want me to register our classes for expectant mothers for you?

45. 每个孕周都有不同的检查。

There are different examinations in different gestational weeks.

46. 您每次来产检都需要检测尿。

You need to take a urine test every time you

come to see your doctor during your pregnancy.

47. 您学会数胎动了吗?

Have you learnt how to count fetal movements?

48. 我来教您如何数胎动。

Let me teach you how to count fetal movements.

49. 28 周后开始测胎动。

Fetal movements can be calculated after 28 weeks.

50. 每天 3 次，每次 1 小时。

You should calculate it 3 times a day, lasting at least one hour each time.

51. 测胎动最好在饭后进行。

Fetal movements should be counted after meal.

52. 测胎动需要左侧卧位。

When you count fetal movements, please keep a left lateral position.

53. 测胎动需要精神集中。

Please concentrate while counting fetal movements.

54. 正常胎动每小时 3～5 次。

Normal frequency of fetal movement is 3～5 times per hour.

55. 如果胎动明显减少（少于 12 小时内 20 次或 1 小时 3 次）。

If the fetal movement decreases much less than normal (20 times within 12 hours or 3 times within 1 hour).

如果胎动突然变得急促。

or if the fetal movement suddenly becomes very rapid.

往往表示缺氧。

it usually indicates the lack of oxygen.

需提高警惕并到急诊就诊。

Please stay alert to that and go to the Emergency Room for further checkup.

56. 孕期的饮食要均衡。

Please keep a balanced diet during your pregnancy.

57. 孕期保持能量充沛。

Please keep energetic during your pregnancy.

58. 每顿饭中均有蛋白质。

Each meal should contain protein.

59. 孕期体重增长需注意。

Pay attention to your weight gaining during pregnancy.

第一孕期（1~12 周）：增长 1~2kg。

In the first trimester of pregnancy (1~12weeks), you can gain 1 to 2kg.

第二、三孕期（13～40 周）＜ 0.5 千克／周。

In the second and third trimesters of pregnancy, you can gain less than 0.5kg per week.

整个孕周体重增长 12～15kg。

During the whole pregnancy, an expectant mother could gain between 12 to 15kg.

60. 孕期锻炼以低强度运动为宜。

During your pregnancy, it's suitable to do some low-intensity physical exercises.

61. 在医生指导下，充分热身后进行锻炼。

Under the guidance of your doctor, do exercises after sufficient warming up.

62. 孕期中游泳或步行均可。

It's suitable to swim or walk during pregnancy.

63. 如果发现破水，要及时来医院就诊。

If your water breaks, please come to the hospital right away.

64. 在孕 12 周时，会做超声检查，测量颈部透明带厚度（NT）。

In the 12th week of the pregnancy, you need to take an ultrasound test to measure nuchal translucency (NT).

65. 15 周或 16 周就可以听到胎心了。

In the 15th or the 16th week of the pregnancy, it's possible to hear fetal heart sound.

66. 常规产检很重要。

Regular antenatal examination is very important.

67. 要按时进行产检。

Please come to take antenatal examinations on time.

68. 如有并发症，请及时就诊于相关科室。

If you have any complications, please come to the hospital and consult relative specialties.

69. 要做好生产准备。

Please be prepared for your childbirth.

70. 准备好妈妈用物，包括卫生巾、吸奶器、洗漱用品、护垫等。

Please prepare all the stuff that a mommy needs, including sanitary napkins, breast pump, toiletries, pads, etc.

71. 宝宝用品包括口水巾、尿裤、奶粉、奶瓶、湿纸巾、浴液、洗发水、润肤露等。

Baby's stuff include saliva towels, diapers, milk powder, feeding bottle, wet tissues, body lotion, shampoo, moisturizer, etc.

妇科巡诊
Making a Round of Visits in Gynecology Department

1. 您在月经期吗?

   Are you in your period now?

2. 您月经正常吗?

   Is your period regular?

3. 月经多长时间来 1 次?

   How often is your period?

4. 月经每次持续多长时间?

   How long does your period last each time?

5. 月经量多吗?

   Is there too much menstrual blood?

6. 平时用卫生护垫吗?

   Do you usually use pads?

7. 这个检查要月经期的第 2 ~ 4 天。

   This examination should be done during the 2nd and 4th day of your period.

8. 月经干净后 4 ~ 7 天再来检查。

   Please come to take the examination 4 to7 days after your period completely finishes.

9. 您预约下次复诊时间了吗？

Have you made an appointment for your next consultation?

10. 您是下腹痛是吗？

Do you have pain in your lower abdomen?

11. 您来月经时痛吗？

Do you feel painful when you are in your period?

12. 医生会给您做简单的妇科检查。

The doctor will give you a simple gynecological examination.

13. 您做过 TCT 检查吗？

Have you taken a TCT test before?

14. 您做过 HPV 检查吗？

Have you taken a HPV test before?

15. 医生让您做阴道镜检查吗？

Did your doctor ask you to take a colposcopy examination?

16. 您需要做术前检查。

You need to take some preoperative examinations.

17. 术前检查需要抽血。

You need to take a blood test for preoperative examination.

牙科巡诊
Making a Round of Visits in Dental Department

1. 一天要刷两次牙。

   Brush your teeth twice a day.

2. 每天刷牙需要 3 分钟才能刷到牙齿所有部位。

   It takes 3 minutes to brush all parts of your teeth every day.

3. 牙刷刷毛与牙龈缘呈 45°角。

   The angle between the toothbrush bristles and the gingival margin should be 45°.

4. 水平颤动牙刷，用适度的力量去除牙菌斑。

   Vibrate the toothbrush horizontally and remove the plague with a modest force.

5. 刷上颌牙，牙刷应向下运动。

   The toothbrush should move downwards when you brush the maxillary teeth.

6. 刷下颌牙，牙刷应向上运动。

   The toothbrush should move upwards when you brush the mandibular teeth.

7. 3 颗牙为一组。

A group consists of 3 teeth.

8. 每组重复刷 10 次左右。

Brush each group for about 10 times.

9. 每次饭后您都应该刷牙或漱口。

You should brush your teeth or rinse your mouth after every meal.

10. 请选择软毛牙刷。

Please select a soft fur toothbrush.

11. 牙刷每 3 个月更换 1 次。

Replace the toothbrush every 3 months.

12. 每次刷牙后应将牙刷清洗干净并甩干。

The brush should be cleaned and dried every time after you use it.

13. 请选择含氟牙膏，正确刷牙。

Please select a fluorine toothpaste and brush your teeth properly.

14. 含氟牙膏有助于预防龋齿。

The fluorine toothpaste can help you prevent the dental caries.

15. 儿童请使用儿童专用牙膏。

Children should use special toothpaste for children.

16. 刷牙水温度适宜在 30～36℃。

The water temperature for teeth brushing is better between 30 ~ 36℃。

17. 切忌几个人用一把牙刷。

Avoid using the same toothbrush among several persons.

18. 每半年检查一次口腔。

Take an oral examination every half a year.

19. 每半年或 1 年口腔洁治 1 次。

Have your teeth cleaned every half a year or a year.

20. 如佩戴活动义齿，应定期使用义齿清洁剂清洗。

If wearing a removable denture, you should clean it with the denture cleaner regularly.

眼科巡诊
Making a Round of Visits in Ophthalmology Department

1. 您查视力了吗？

Have you tested your vision?

2. 您的孩子是早产吗？

Is your child a premature infant?

3. 您今天是来检查眼底的吗？

Do you come to check your fundus today?

4. 您散瞳了吗？

Did you get mydriasis?

5. 您需要测眼压。

You need to measure intraocular pressure.

6. 捂住您的左眼。

Please cover your left eye.

7. 我们要测您的右眼视力。

We are going to test the vision of your right eye.

8. 换过来，捂住您的右眼。

Please cover your right eye.

9. 现在我们来测您的左眼视力。

Now let's test the vision of your left vision.

10. 告诉我这些 E 的指向（上、下、左、右）。

Tell me the directions of these "E" s. (Up, down, left, right).

11. 这行看得清楚吗？

Can you see this line clearly?

12. 那么下一行呢？

What about the next line?

13. 不要使劲压着左眼。否则，查左眼时会受影响。

Don't press your left eye too hard. Or the vision result of your left eye will be affected.

14. 这是您的视力初检结果。

This is the test result of your vision.

耳鼻喉科巡诊
Making a Round of Visits
in E.N.T Department

1. 您的听力下降了是吗?

Do you have hearing loss?

2. 医生是让您测量听力吗?

Did your doctor ask you to take a hearing test?

3. 您的听力测试要在一个特定的检查室进行。

Your hearing test will be done in a specific examination room.

4. 等下,有导医带您去查听力。

Wait a second. Our hospital guide will lead you to take the examination.

5. 是卡鱼刺了吗?

Did a fish bone stick in your throat?

Did you choke on fish bone?

6. 医生要给您检查咽喉。

The doctor will check your throat.

7. 您放松,配合一下。

Please relax and do as what the doctor tell you.

8. 我先给您喷一点麻药在咽部。再按着医生教您的方法做。

   I will spray some anesthetic on your throat. Then follow the doctor's lead.

9. 医生会为您做鼻咽镜的检查。

   Your doctor will perform a nasopharyngoscopy for you.

10. 这是医生给您开的点耳朵里的药。

    Here is the ear drop prescribed by your doctor for you.

11. 等耳朵里的耵聍出来了，再来医院医生给您冲洗。

    Please wait for the earwax to come out, Then come to the hospital and the doctor will rinse your ear for you.

12. 这是治疗咽炎的药。

    This is the medicine for your pharyngitis.

13. 您要按时吃药。

    Please take your medicine on time.

四、

预　　约
Appointment

门诊预约
Outpatient Appointment

1. 请问您需要预约哪个医生？

   Which doctor do you want to make an appointment with?

2. 请问您哪里不舒服？我们为您选择合适的医生。

   How do you feel? We will recommend a doctor for you.

3. 对不起，某某医生已经预约满了，您可以选择另一位专家或更改您的预约时间吗？

   Sorry, Dr. X is fully booked on that day. Could you please choose another specialist or change your appointment time?

4. 我们可以根据您及医生合适的时间，为您特约某某医生。

   According to your time and the doctor's schedule, we will make an appointment with Dr. X for you.

5. 已为您预约好了周四上午九点的某某医生。

   We have made an appointment for you with Dr. X at 9 o'clock on Thursday morning.

6. 明天上午没有神经科，下午有，可以吗？

There is no neurologists available tomorrow morning. Is it OK for you to see a neurologist tomorrow afternoon?

7. 某某医生没有常规门诊，我们可以为您专门预约专科医生。

Dr. X doesn't have a regular outpatient service, but we can make a specialist appointment for you.

8. 请问您要预约哪位医生？

Which specialist would you like to consult?

9. 请问您要预约哪个科？

Which department do you want to make an appointment with?

10. 第一次就诊请记得携带身份证原件办理就诊卡。

In your first-time visit to our hospital, please take your personal ID card to apply for a Hospital ID card.

11. 您选择的科室没有常规门诊，我们可以给您专门预约专科医生。

There is no available regular outpatient service of that department, but we can make a specialist appointment for you.

12. 做某些检查需要先挂某科的号。

If you want to take some examination, you should register that department first.

13. 预约好了，7月6号周二上午十点的心内科。请您准时就诊。

We have made an appointment for you: Cardiology, 10 am on July 6th, Tuesday. Please come to the hospital on time.

14. 若来不了，请您至少提前一天致电取消。

If you cannot show up on the consulting day, please call us to cancel your appointment at least one day before.

抽血
Blood Drawing

1. 您最好明天早上再来，因为这个血液检查需要空腹。

You'd better come tomorrow morning, because this blood test needs fasting.

2. 该项血液检查有严格的时间要求。

This blood test has rigorous time requirement.

请您明天早上8点钟准时来抽血。

Please come to the hospital for blood drawing at

8 o'clock tomorrow morning.

3. 该项血液检查有特殊要求。

This blood test has special requirements.

抽血前需要站立 1 小时。

You need to stand for 1 hour before the blood drawing.

不能蹲，不能倚靠，并在抽血过程中也需要站立。

No squatting or leaning. You also need to stand during the blood drawing.

4. 妇科激素这项抽血检查医生有没有告诉您有月经期的要求？

This blood test is related to gynecological hormone. Has your doctor told you whether this test has the requirement of menstrual period?

尿标本
Urine Sample

1. 该项尿沉渣检查有时间的要求。

Urinary sediment test has time requirement.

2. 请您工作日上午 10 点半之前将标本留好送检。

Please send your urine sample for test before 10:30 am on workdays.

神经科
Neurology Department

1. 肌电图检查需到 **xxxxx** 处划价后交费再预约时间进行检查；两天后出结果。

   If you need to take an electromyography(EMG), please go to XXXXX to have your prescription priced, then pay the fee and come back to make an appointment for the test; you can get the test result in two days.

2. 脑电图在位于 **xxxxx** 的脑电图室预约检查。

   You need to make an appointment of Electroencephalography (EEG) in EEG Room, which is located at XXXXX.

   检查前一天晚上需洗头并不能喷任何物品。

   Please wash your hair the night before the test and avoid spaying anything on your hair.

3. 儿科脑电图在位于 **xxxxx** 的实验室。

   Pediatric EEG is in Pediatric Lab, which is at XXXXX.

4. 经颅多普勒（**TCD**）检查在 **xxxxx** 处做。

   TCD test examination room is located at XXXXX.

内分泌科
Endocrinology Department

1. 如需注射胰岛素针，请携带就诊卡和导诊单到 xxxxx 处护士站取。

   To get insulin needles, please go to the Nurse Station which is located at XXXXX with your Hospital ID Card and Examination Guide Sheet.

2. 如果您需要预约甲状腺 FNAB，请到 xxxxx 处。

   If you need to make an appointment of Thyroid FNAB, please go to XXXXX.

变态反应科
Allergy Department

1. 如需做肺功能检查，请持就诊卡前往 xxxxx 处做。

   If you need to take a pulmonary function test, please go to XXXXX with your Hospital ID Card.

2. 如果您需要做皮肤测试，请持就诊卡前往 xxxxx 处做。

If you need to take a skin test, please go to XXXXX with your Hospital ID Card.

呼吸内科
Department of
Respiratory Medicine

1. 通气＋可逆、一氧化碳检查在肺功能室做，做时患者需要提供身高、体重、出生日期。

   Ventilation function test + airway reversibility and carbon monoxide test can be done in Lung Function Test Room. Patients need to provide the information of their height, weight and birth date.

   通气＋可逆检查当时即可出结果，一氧化碳检查两个工作日后出结果。

   For the former two tests, patients can get the results immediately after the test; for the last one, patients can get the result two days after the examination.

2. 呼吸睡眠暂停检测需在 xxxxx 处预约。

   If you need to take sleep apnea test, please make an appointment at XXXXX.

3．检查时需自行准备小便器。

Please prepare a urinal before taking this examination.

消化科
Department of Gastroenterology

1．数字胃肠造影检查在 xxxxx 处做。

Digital radiography of the gastrointestinal track can be done at XXXXX.

两个工作日后在 xxxxx 处取结果。

Patients can get the results at XXXXX after two workdays.

2．C^{13}、C^{14} 检查前，患者需要在 xxxxx 处取得条码。

Before taking C^{13} (Carbon 13), C^{14} (Carbon 14) tests, patients need to get the barcode at XXXXX.

在 xxxxx 处检查，30 分钟出结果。

The tests will be done at XXXXX and patients can get the results after 30 minutes.

儿科
Pediatrics Department

1. 儿科头颅 B 超在 xxxxx 处预约。

   To take pediatric cranial ultrasound, you need to make an appointment at XXXXX.

   这项检查每周四才能做。

   The test is scheduled on every Thursday.

2. 胎儿核磁在 xxxxx 处预约。

   For fetal MRI test, you need to make an appointment at XXXXX.

   请按照预约好的时间、地点进行检查。

   Take the examination at the appointed time and place please.

眼科
Ophthalmology Department

1. 眼科 OCT、视野、眼科超声检查在位于 xxxxx 处的眼科检查室做。

   Patients can take the OCT test, perimetry and ophthalmic ultrasound test in the Ophthalmic

Examination Room which is located at XXXXX.

2. 眼科部分其他检查在 xxxxx 处预约及检查。

Some other ophthalmic tests can be scheduled and done at XXXXX.

皮肤科
Dermatology Department

1. 药物面膜需携带就诊卡、导诊单到 xxxxx 处取；面膜需要冷藏。

To get medical facial masks, you should go to XXXXX with your Hospital ID Card and Examination Guide; the facial masks need to be refrigerated.

2. 冷冻治疗需到 xxxxx 处做。

For cryotherapy, you should go to XXXXX.

3. 治疗时间为：周一、周五全天，二、三、四上午。

Treatment Time: Full day every Monday and Friday, only morning every Tuesday, Wednesday and Thursday.

心内科
Cardiology Department

1. 心电图检查在就诊楼层治疗室做。

   ECG can be done at the treatment room on the same floor where you see your doctor.

   心内科、普通内科的心电图检查直接将报告交至患者。

   The ECG reports from Cardiology and Internal Medicine will be given to you immediately.

   妇产科心电图检查，有大病历者的报告自动回大病历。

   The ECG reports of OBS and GYN will be sent back to your Medical Record if you have one.

   无大病历者可到妇科护士站取心电图检查结果。

   Otherwise the reports will be sent to the Nurse Station of GYN.

   其他科室需 3 个工作日后到 xxxxx 处取结果。

   For ECG prescribed by other specialties, patients can get the report at XXXXX after three workdays.

2. 动态心电图需到 xxxxx 处预约；每周一、三、四、五下午在 xxxxx 处做检查。

You can make an appointment of dynamic ECG at XXXXX. You can have the Dynamic ECG test at XXXXX on the afternoon of every Monday, Wednesday, Thursday, and Friday.

3. 平板需在 xxxxx 处预约；1 个工作日后出结果。

For the test of treadmill exercise, you need to make an appointment at XXXXX. And you can get the report one workday after the test is done.

骨科
Orthopedics Department

1. 骨密度检查需携带导诊单到 xxxxx 处换检查单。

For Bone Mineral Density (BMD) test, please go to XXXXX to get your Examination Note with your Examination Guide.

换完检查单后请安静等候检查。

After getting the Examination Note, please wait for the examination quietly.

时间为周一至周五早 8 点 ~ 11 点。

The time is 8:00am ~ 11:00am from Monday to Friday.

2. 磁共振（MRI）检查均需携带就诊卡、导诊单到

xxxxx 处预约。

For any Magnetic Resonance Imaging (MRI) test, please make an appointment at XXXXX with your Hospital ID Card and Examination Guide.

然后按照预约时间、地点去检查。

Then take the examination according to the appointed time and place.

需仔细阅读检查须知注意事项。

Please read the examination notice carefully.

增强 MRI 需取药，并有家属陪同。

For enhanced MRI, you need to pick up medicine first and get accompanied by your families.

3. CT、CTU、CTA 在 xxxxx 处预约和检查。

For CT, CTU, CTA Scan, you need to make an appointment and take the test at XXXXX.

普通 CT 当日可做。

For regular CT scan, you can do it on the same day of seeing your doctor.

增强 CT 需带药，家属陪同。

For enhanced CT, you need to take the medicine and get accompanied by your families.

低剂量 CT 在外科楼地下一层做。

For low-dose CT, you need to take it on the underground floor of the Surgical Building.

耳鼻喉科
Otorhinolaryngology
(ENT) Department

1. 喉镜在 xxxxx 处检查。

   Laryngoscope inspection is taken at XXXXX.

2. 助听器在 xxxxx 处配做。

   If you need hearing aid, please go to XXXXX.

3. 听力等其他耳鼻喉科检查都在 xxxxx 处预约及检查。

   For hearing and other E.N.T tests, you need to make an appointment and take the tests at XXXXX.

其他
Others

1. 精液检查需在相应楼层取血室打条码；然后再到 xxxxx 处预约及检查。

   For semen examination, you need to get the bar

code in the Blood Drawing Room on the same floor of seeing your doctor. Then schedule and take your examination at XXXXX.

2. PET/CT 在 xxxxx 处预约；检查当日不能做其他任何检查。

For PET/CT scanning, you need to make an appointment at XXXXX. On the examination day, you are not allowed to take any other examinations.

请仔细阅读检查注意事项，请按照预约好的时间和地点做检查。

Please read the examination notice carefully and take the examination at the appointed time and place.

3. 碘实验在 xxxxx 处预约；检查在 xxxxx 处做。

For Iodine Test, you need to make an appointment at XXXXX; You can take the test at XXXXX.

五、

注意事项
Notice

胃肠镜检查前注意事项
Tips before Gastroscopy/ Colonoscopy

1. 胃镜检查前 1 日的晚餐要在 9：00pm 前用完；进食量要少于平常。

   For gastroscopy examinees, please have dinner before 21:00 the day before and eat less than usual.

2. 检查当日不吃早餐，也不要喝水。

   Don't have breakfast or drink water on the examination day.

3. 无痛胃镜检查前 1 日，夜间 midnight 后严格禁食禁水。

   For painless gastroscopy examinees, please take no food or water after 24:00 the day before examination.

4. 结肠镜检查前 3 日，禁食不易消化的食物（蔬菜、水果等纤维或种子较多的食物）。

   For colonoscopy examinees, please don't eat any indigestible foods (vegetable, fruit or other food which contain a lot of fiber or seeds) 3 days before the examination.

5. 普通结肠镜检查前 1 日，一定要在 7：00 pm 前用完晚餐。

For general colonoscopy examinees, please have dinner before 19:00 the day before.

6. 餐后不可进食，但可喝水。

After dinner, only water is allowed.

7. 上午检查者前 1 日晚餐后遵照医嘱饮用 2 升清肠液；上午检查前 3 ~ 4 小时再饮 1 升清肠液。

If you have a colonoscopy in the morning, please follow the doctor's order to drink 2 liters of intestine-rinsing fluid after having dinner the day before. And drink another 1 liter 3 ~ 4 hours before the examination.

8. 无痛检查者前 1 天晚餐后，遵照医嘱饮 3L 清肠液，夜间 midnight 后严格禁食禁水。

For painless colonoscopy examines, please drink 3 liters of intestine-rinsing fluid after having dinner the day before, and no food or water is allowed after midnight.

9. 胃镜和结肠镜检查前 1 周，均需要停用阿司匹林、波立维（氯吡格雷）、华法林等抗凝药物。

Before having a gastroscopy or colonoscopy,

please stop taking aspirin, Plavix (clopidogrel), warfarin or other anticoagulants 1 week before the examination.

停药或药物调整，请务必在专业医师指导下进行。

Please stop or adjust the taking of anticoagulants under the guidance of your doctor.

10. 检查当日需有一位直系亲属陪同，以备检查中签字。

Please have your family accompany you on the examination day in case there is a need of signing.

11. 检查前需完成麻醉科会诊，并完成血液感染4项检查。

Please consult an anesthesiologist and complete 4 blood infection tests before examination.

12. 根据检查中操作及麻醉的实际需要，检查后需补交费用。

Pay the fees after the examination according to the real practice and dosage of anesthesia used.

13. 如需更改预约时间，请拨打国际医疗部门诊电话 xxxxx。

If you want to change your appointment time,

please call XXXXX in advance.

胃镜检查小贴士
Tips for Gastroscopy

1. 请脱掉上衣、眼镜、活动性假牙及皮带等，尽可能让自己感到舒适。

   Please take off your coat, glasses, removable denture and belt. Keep yourself as comfortable as possible.

2. 为了更容易地吞下内镜，需要在检查前服用药物来进行喉部麻醉。

   To help you swallow the gastroscope, you need to take some medicine to get laryngeal anesthesia before the examination.

3. 请含服于喉部 2 分钟，然后咽下。

   Please hold the medicine around your throat for 2 minutes and then swallow it.

   无痛检查者请忽略。

   Examinees of painless gastroscopy please ignore this.

   内镜通过咽喉时会有不适感；内镜通过咽喉后，安静地呼吸（鼻子吸气，嘴呼气）。

When the gastroscope go through your throat, it may feel uncomfortable. Try to breathe quietly (inhale with nose and exhale with mouth).

尽量放松。

Relax yourself.

不要吞咽口腔分泌物，让其顺嘴角自然流到袋子里。

Don't swallow the oral secretion, and just let it flow naturally into the bag.

检查过程需要几分钟（无痛检查者请忽略）。

The whole exam ination only takes several minutes. (Examinees of painless gastroscopy please ignore this).

4. 因麻药有残留作用，检查 1 小时后再进食。

Because of the residual effect of anesthetic, please eat food at least 1 hour after the examination.

避免过烫、粗硬和刺激性食物。

Don't take spicy, hot, hard or excitant food.

若接受无痛内镜检查的患者，检查后请在恢复室休息 30 分钟到 1 个小时。

Examinees of painless gastroscopy need to rest for 30mins to 1h in Recovery Room.

检查当日不要驾车。

Don't drive on your examination day.

结肠镜肠道准备说明
Introduction of the Intestinal Preparation for Colonoscopy

1. 饮食要求：检查的前两天开始少渣饮食。

   Diet Requirements: Patients need to start a low-residue diet two days before the examination.

   如：稀粥、烂面条、蛋羹、藕粉、米糊等。

   You can choose thin porridge, overcooked noodles, egg custard, lotus root starch, rice paste, etc.

   不要进食蔬菜和水果。

   Do not eat vegetables or fruits.

   检查当天应禁食，但可以喝糖水。

   On the examination day, you can only take sugar water.

   麻醉肠镜者术前 6 小时禁食水。

   For colonoscopy with anesthesia, you need to fast for 6 hours before the examination.

2. 服用和爽（可根据具体药物替换）上午检查者：检查前日晚餐后禁食（可以饮水）。

If your examination is to be taken in the morning: For patients who choose Heshuang (this intestinal medicine can be replaced) for intestinal cleaning, keep fasting after dinner (drinking water is available) the night before the examination.

晚餐后3小时开始服用和爽。

Start to drink Heshuang 3 hours after dinner.

下午检查者：检查当日禁食（可以饮水）。

If your examination is to be taken in the afternoon: Keep fasting on the examination day (drinking water is available).

早晨8点开始服用和爽。

Start to drink Heshuang at 8:00 am.

如有严重腹胀或不适。

If severe bloating or discomfort appears.

可放慢服用速度或暂停服药。

Please slow down the speed of drinking Heshuang or suspend it.

症状消除后再继续服用。

And continue to drink it after the symptoms disappear.

3. 和爽配制及服用方法。

Prepare and drink Heshuang solution.

将 3 袋和爽加凉开水配成 3000ml 的溶液。

Blend 3 bags of Heshuang with cold boiled water, making 3000ml solution.

在 2 小时内服用完。

Finish drinking the solution within 2 hours.

在服用过程中请一定要来回走动或轻揉腹部，以保证良好的清肠效果。

When drinking, keep walking around or rubbing your abdomen gently so that the intestine-rinsing fluid can work effectively.

多数情况下，服药 1 小时左右开始第一次排便。

Most likely, you will defecate for the first time in about 1 hour after drinking the solution.

在排便约 5 ~ 8 次后，当排出物为无色或黄色透明水样便时，肠道准备结束。

After defecating for 5 ~ 8 times, your stool becomes water or yellow transparent liquid and this means that intestinal preparation is done.

如最后一次排出物为有形便或渣便。

For the last time you defecate, if there is still residue in the stool.

则需加服和爽，直至排出物为无色或黄色透明水样便。

You need to drink more Heshuang solution until your stool becomes water or yellow transparent liquid.

但总量不得超过 4000ml。

But please notice that the overall volume of Heshuang solution to drink should be less than 4000ml.

4. 选择硫酸镁清洗肠道的患者。

For patients who choose magnesium sulfate for intestinal cleaning.

提前 3 天开始每晚各服酚酞两片，连服两晚，检查前晚不吃。

Start to take two tablets of phenolphthalein each night for 2 consecutive days three days before the examination, but take no phenolphthalein tablet the night before the examination.

上午检查者前一天早上 8 点喝硫酸镁 1 瓶，之后半小时内喝约 2000ml 白开水（5 磅暖瓶一暖瓶）。

If the examination is to be taken in the morning: you need to drink a bottle of magnesium sulfate liquid at 8:00am the day before the examination, and finish drinking 2000ml of cold boiled water within half an hour (A bottle means 5 pounds of liquid).

晚上 7 点再喝硫酸镁 1 瓶，之后半小时内喝约 2000ml 白开水。

Drink another bottle of magnesium sulfate liquid at 7:00pm that evening, and finish drinking 2000ml of cold boiled water within half an hour.

下午检查者当天早上 6 点硫酸镁 1 瓶，之后半小时内喝约 2000ml 白开水。

If the examination is in the afternoon: you need to drink a bottle of magnesium sulfate liquid at 6:00am on the examination day, and finish drinking 2000ml of cold boiled water within half an hour.

上午 11 点再喝硫酸镁 1 瓶。

Drink another bottle of magnesium sulfate liquid at 11:00am.

之后半小时内喝约 2000ml 白开水。

Finish drinking 2000ml of cold boiled water within half an hour.

* 腹泻严重者，请及时补充饮水，直至解出清水样便为止。

*If you have severe diarrhea, please drink water

timely until your stool becomes water or yellow transparent liquid.

5. 行麻醉肠镜患者肠道准备均按上午检查的程序进行。

For colonoscopy patients with anesthesia, you need to prepare your intestine according to the requirements of morning examination.

检查前 6 小时严格禁食水。

Keep fasting for 6 hours before the examination.

6. 奥布卡因凝胶（纸盒的药）检查当天带着，检查时使用。

Please remember to bring Oxybuprocaine Hydrochloride Gel (medicine in paper box) on the examination day for the usage during the examination.

结肠镜检查小贴士
Tips for Colonoscopy

1. 穿检查裤时开裆向后，不穿内衣。

When putting on the split examination pants, please keep the split at your back. Take off your underwear.

在检查台上左侧卧位，尽量放松。

Lie on your left side on the examination table and relax as much as you can.

2. 为了更好地观察结肠，检查过程中医生可能会要求您从左侧卧位变为右侧卧位或仰卧位。

For better observation results, doctors may ask you to change to right lateral position or supine position from left lateral position.

仰卧位时您的右腿要放在左腿上（"跷二郎腿"）。

When you lie on your back, please put your right leg on your left one.

（无痛检查者请忽略）。

(Examinees of painless gastroscopy please ignore this).

3. 如果做了内镜下息肉切除手术，为了防止出血，手术后3日内需进流食。

If polypectomy is conducted during the exam, to prevent bleeding, please drink fluids within 3 days after the exam.

1周内避免运动、旅行及出差。

Avoid physical exercise or travelling within 1 week.

若有大出血、腹痛等表现，请及时返院复诊。

If there appears a massive hemorrhage or stomachache, please return to the hospital timely for further consultation.

4. 若接受的是无痛内镜检查，因麻药残留作用，检查后请在恢复室休息 30 分钟到 1 个小时。

Patients who take painless colonoscopy need to rest for 30mins-1h in the Recovery Room owing to the residual effect of anesthetic.

检查当日不要驾车。

Don't drive on your examination day.

胃镜 / 直结肠镜检查报告
Report of Gastroscopy/Colonoscopy

1. 内镜检查完成后，检查医生当时就会给您出镜下所见报告。

When the gastroscopy/colonoscopy is done, your examination doctors will give you your report.

报告原件保存在您的大病历内，由我院为您永久保存。

The original one will be put in your Medical

Record, which will be stored in our hospital.

您下次来我院就诊时，大病历会由医院专人送至相应科室。

When you come to see a doctor in our hospital, your Medical Record will be handed to your doctor.

如果您想保存这份报告，可以用手机拍照或复印。

You can take a photo or make a hard copy.

2. 活检是医师根据您的病情在检查时取的小块组织。

Biopsy refers to the tissue removed from a patient by the doctor as needed.

送到病理科做进一步检查。

And it will be sent to Pathology for further examination.

门诊患者需持就诊卡交化验费。

For outpatients, you need to pay the bills for biopsy with your Hospital ID Card.

5~7个工作日出报告，报告回大病历内。

The biopsy result will be put into your Medical Record after 5 to 7 workdays.

牙线使用小贴士
Tips for Dental floss

1. 牙线是用来清洁牙间隙的工具。

   The dental floss is a tool used to clean teeth.

2. 从牙线盒里拉出约 25cm 长的牙线。

   Pull out 25cm of dental floss from the dental floss box.

3. 将牙线的两端分别绕在两手的中指上。

   Wind both ends of the dental floss around both middle fingers respectively.

4. 两个中指中留出 5cm 长牙线。

   Keep 5cm of dental floss between two middle fingers.

5. 通过手指的牵位来控制牙线。

   Control the dental floss by the holding position of fingers.

6. 一个手指在口内，一个手指在口外。

   One middle finger is in the mouth and the other one is out.

7. 通过牙线的滑动，将食物嵌渣带出。

   Bring the food residues out by sliding the dental

floss.

8. 每个牙面均需上下摩擦。

Each tooth surface needs to be rubbed up and down.

9. 将牙线贴紧牙面变成 C 形。

Make the dental floss close to the tooth surface and turn to C-shape.

10. 用同样的方法，清洗全口牙齿。

Clean all the teeth in the mouth in the same way.

11. 牙线使用后需用清水漱口。

Rinse your mouth with clean water after using the dental floss.

牙科治疗后注意事项
Tips for Dental Posttreatment

1. 拔牙后：

After tooth extraction：

纱球 30 ~ 40 分钟后吐掉。

Spit out the yarn ball after 30 ~ 40 minutes.

拔牙当天不刷牙。

Don't brush your teeth on the day of tooth extraction.

拔牙当日勿食过热饮食，可食用凉饮食。

Don't eat hot food on the day of tooth extraction, but cold food is OK.

不要用舌头舔牙窝。

Don't lick the extraction socket.

2. 补牙后：

After the dental filling:

补牙当天，避免用患牙侧咀嚼食物。

Don't use the same side with the dental filling to eat on the day of the dental filling.

补牙后2小时内不要用患牙吃东西。

Don't use the affected tooth to eat something after the dental filling within 2 hours.

补牙当天不吃过黏过硬的食物。

Don't eat sticky or hard foods on the day of the dental filling.

3. 修复义齿类注意事项：

Notice for denture use：

饭后应将活动义齿取下。用冷水冲洗后再戴上。

The denture should be removed after a meal. Wash it with cold water and then put it on.

睡觉时应将义齿摘下。

The denture should be taken off when you go to bed.

义齿在清洁后浸泡于冷水后。

The denture should be soaked in cold water after cleaning.

每周用义齿清洁药片彻底清洁 1～2 次。

The denture should be deep cleaned regularly with the denture cleanser for 1～2 times.

产科
Obstetrics

1. 口服葡萄糖耐量试验。

   Oral Glucose Tolerance Test (OGTT).

√ 50g 葡萄糖耐量试验方法：

   50g OGTT:

   检查当日 0 点后禁食禁水。

   Keep fasting after 0:00am on the test day.

   早 8 点携带葡萄糖粉及就诊卡到取血室。

   Bring your glucose powder and Hospital ID Card to the Blood Drawing Room by 8:00am on the test day.

由护士溶解糖粉后，5 分钟之内喝下去。

The nurse will help you dissolve the glucose powder, and you need to finish drinking it within 5 minutes.

并从喝的第一口开始计时，1 小时抽血。

Count from the first sip, and get your blood drawn after 1 hour.

并注意在此期间不要有频繁或剧烈的活动，最好静坐休息，以免影响结果的准确。

Please sit and wait quietly and avoid strenuous exercises, otherwise the test result will be affected.

1 个工作日后，自助打印结果。

You will get your OGTT result after 1 workday. The report could be printed on the self-service machine.

血糖正常范围 <7.8mmol/L。

FYI, Normal Blood Glucose: <7.8mmol/L.

√ 75g 葡萄糖耐量试验方法：

75g OGTT:

试验前连续 3 天正常体力活动、正常饮食。

Do regular physical activities and keep a normal diet for three days before the test.

检查前一日晚 10 点后禁食禁水。

Keep fasting after 10:00pm the night before the test.

早 8 点携带葡萄糖粉及就诊卡到取血室。

Bring your glucose powder and Hospital ID Card to the Blood Drawing Room by 8:00am on the test day.

先抽血测空腹血糖（最迟不超过上午 9 点）。

First, the nurse will draw your blood for fasting-blood glucose (before 9:00am).

由护士溶解糖粉后，5 分钟之内喝下去。

The nurse will help you dissolve the glucose powder, and you need to finish drinking it within 5minutes.

并从喝的第一口开始计时，于服糖后 1 小时、2 小时分别抽血测血糖。

Count from the first sip, and get your blood drawn twice after 1hour and 2hours respectively.

并注意在此期间不要有频繁或剧烈的活动，最好静坐休息，以免影响结果的准确。

Please sit and wait quietly and avoid strenuous exercises, or the test result will be affected.

1 个工作日后，自助打印结果。

You will get your OGTT result after 1 workday. The report could be printed on the self-service machine.

血糖正常范围：

Normal Blood Glucose:

空腹 <5.1mmol/L，1 小时 <10.0mmol/L，2 小时 <8.5mmol/L.

Fasting-blood glucose <5.1mmol/L, 1hour blood glucose<10.0 mmol/L, 2hour blood glucose<8.5 mmol/L.

有任何一项指标超标，请及时就诊。

If any indicator exceeds the normal limit, please consult a doctor immediately.

2. 胎动的监测。

Monitoring of Fetal Movements.

28 周后开始监测胎动。

Expectant moms can start to monitor fetal movements after 28 weeks into pregnancy.

每天 3 次，每次 1 小时。

You can do the monitoring three times a day, and 1 hour each time.

宜饭后进行，左侧卧位，精神集中。

Do it after meals. Keep a left lateral position and

focus on the monitoring.

正常胎动每小时至少 3～5 次。

Normally, 3 to 5 fetal movements will appear each hour.

如胎动明显减少（12 小时内少于 20 次或 1 小时内胎动少于 3 次）或胎动突然变得急促，往往表示胎儿缺氧。

If the fetal movements decrease sharply (less than 20 times within 12 hours or less than 3 times within 1 hour) or become fast suddenly, it usually indicates the fetus is in oxygen shortage.

孕妇不可掉以轻心，应到急诊就诊。

Expectant moms should pay close attention to this and go to the Emergency Room immediately.

3. 饮食与体重。

Diet and Weight.

孕期饮食原则：全面、均衡摄取营养；保持能量充沛，每顿饭或加餐中均有蛋白质（如蛋、禽类、鱼）、碳水化合物（蔬菜、水果、谷物）、健康的脂肪（橄榄油或坚果）。

Prenatal diet principles: keep a comprehensive and balanced diet; keep energetic, each meal and extra meal should contain protein (such as eggs, poultry, fish), carbon dioxide (such as vegetable, fruit, grain), and healthy fat (such as olive oil and nut).

孕期体重增长：第一孕期（1~12周）：1~2kg。

Weight gain during pregnancy: first trimester (1 ~ 12 weeks): 1 ~ 2 kg.

第二~三孕期（13~40周）：< 0.5 千克 / 周。

The second and third trimesters (13 ~ 40weeks): < 0.5kg/week.

整个孕期：12~15kg。

The whole pregnancy: 12 ~ 15kg.

4. 乳房护理。

Breast Care.

孕期选用棉质的、大小合适的胸罩。

During the pregnancy, please wear cotton sizable bras.

怀孕 6 个月后，每天用湿毛巾擦拭乳头 1 次。

After being pregnant for 6 months, please wipe your nipples with wet towel once a day.

擦洗时用力应均匀，柔和，勿伤皮肤。

Wipe them gently and equally, avoiding hurting your skin.

经常擦洗可使乳头坚韧，喂奶时不易破裂。

Wiping can help to make nipples strong and they won't break easily when breast feeding.

勿用肥皂，如有宫缩应暂停刺激乳房。

Do not use soap when wiping; if there appears UC (uterine contraction), please stop stimulating your breasts.

5. 孕期锻炼。

Exercise during Pregnancy.

锻炼原则：以低强度有氧运动为宜，并遵守医生的指导。

Workout principles: please choose low intensity cardio activity and follow your doctor's instruction.

充分热身后进行锻炼，如缩肛锻炼（**Kegel** 锻炼）、游泳、步行等。

An adequate warming up is necessary before doing the exercises. Kegel exercise, swimming, and jogging are recommended.

运动量不应大于孕前的标准。

The amount of exercise should be less than that before the pregnancy.

6. 临产预兆。

Signs of Labor.

见红：在分娩发动前 24～48 小时，因宫颈口附近的胎膜与该处的子宫壁分离；毛细血管破裂经阴道排出少量血液，与宫颈管内的黏液栓相混排出。

Bleeding Show: 24 ~ 48 hours before childbirth, fetal membranes near the cervix get separated from the uterus wall, which causes the breaking of blood capillaries, and as a result, a small amount of blood or blood-tinged mucus will be excreted through the vagina.

这种现象称为见红。

This phenomenon is called bloody show.

见红是分娩即将开始的比较可靠征象。

Bloody show is a reliable sign for the beginning of childbirth.

宫缩：宫缩间隔 5 ~ 6 分钟，持续 30 秒。

Uterine Contraction (UC)：UC has an interval of 5 ~ 6 minutes and each one lasts for around 30 seconds.

间隔时间越来越短。

The interval will become shorter and shorter.

子宫一阵阵发硬，并疼痛或腰酸，意味着分娩马上要开始。

Your uterus will become hard now with pain or

soreness of waist, and this means that childbirth will start very soon.

这时宝宝在说"妈妈，我要出来了！"

The baby is saying "Mommy, I'm getting out!"

这时，你应该准备来医院了。

This is when you should come to the hospital.

破水：指羊膜腔破裂羊水流出的现象。

Membrane rupture means that the membrane breaks and water comes out.

正常的生产是在子宫口开大的过程中或子宫口开全、胎儿进入产道时才会开始破水。

Normally, the water breaks when the uterine orifice opens gradually or uterine orifice opens completely and fetus has entered birth canal.

如果感觉在出现阵痛前有水从阴道流出，可能是早期破水，应到医院检查，及时治疗。

If water comes out through the vagina before labor pain, there may appear premature rupture and you need go to the hospital for examination and timely treatment.

否则可能会引起细菌感染，或发生脐带掉入阴道内（脐带脱垂）的情况，导致胎儿死亡。

It may cause infection and even fetal death if

umbilical cord falls into your vagina (the prolapse of cord).

7. 急诊入院

Emergency Hospitalization

当您孕期出现宫缩、破水、胎动异常、出血等任何紧急情况时，请及时到急诊就诊。

If there appears uterine contraction, membrane rupture, abnormal fetal movement, bloody show and other urgent conditions, please come to the Emergency Room.

急诊位于 **xxxxx** 处，全天 24 小时接诊。

Emergency Room is located at XXXXX, and it provides 24-hour services.

急诊电话: **xxxxx**

Emergency Phone: XXXXX

8. 入院准备

Preparation for Hospitalization

物品的准备:

Goods need to be prepared:

妈妈: 卫生巾、合适内裤、吸奶器;

For mom: sanitary napkins, sizable underpants, breast pump;

婴儿: 尿裤、奶瓶、奶粉、湿纸巾、浴液、护臀霜、洗发水、润肤霜、消毒奶瓶用具。

For baby: diapers, milk bottle, milk powder, wet tissue, baby lotion, diaper rash cream, shampoo, body cream, a bottle sterilizer.

常规入院：产检时由门诊医生开具住院证。

Regular Hospitalization: Your obstetrician will issue a hospitalization certification to you during the prenatal examination.

得到病房医生通知后，请携带好就诊卡和押金到 xxxxx 处办理住院手续。

When the ward doctor calls you and tells you the date of hospitalization, please bring your Hospital ID Card and advance deposit, go to XXXXX to complete formalities for admission.

产科门诊电话：xxxxx

Obstetrics Clinic: XXXXX

全体医务人员祝您及家人
身体健康！天天开心！

All Medical Workers Wish
You and Your Family
Healthiness and Happiness!